Tai Chi Classics
Wang Zongyue Treatise
Decoded

The Science and Practice of Manipulating Force

學力而有為

Reference Manual

Dr. John K. Fung

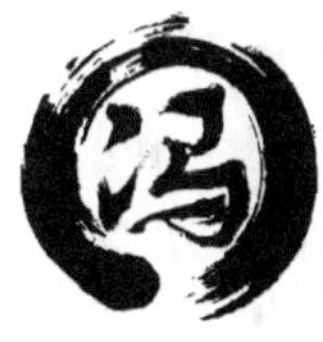

Copyright Information

Front cover:

The stone relief featured on the front cover is one of two
that were stolen from a Buddhist monastery at Taiyuan in
Shanxi Province, northern China, during the winter of
1927. Arrived in 1928 along with the architectural
building, it has been installed in The Dayton Art Institute
ever since.

The panel shows two dragons flying above the churning
water, guarding a pearl that represents the Yin and Yang
manifesting from the undifferentiated chaos, guarding the
pearl of Taiji, the grand ultimate. The dragons also
represent the duality of power and compassion, authority
and benevolence, knowledge and wisdom, Gang and Rou.

The dynamic carving and diagonal composition indicate a
date from the Ming period (1368-1644). The massive
scale of the panel, as well as the five-clawed dragon
design, suggests that these panels are similar to the large
dragon panels on the stairs of one of the three greatest
royal halls in Beijing's Imperial Palace, which was created
by the Ming court in the early fifteenth century.

The image is made public under the Creative Commons
CC0 1.0 Universal Public Domain Dedication.

Dedicated to my two teachers

The Late Grandmaster Wei Shuren

Imperial Yang Tai Chi, Beijing

魏樹人師父

楊式太極拳 北京

and

The Late Master Leung Wunzi

Kulo Wing Chun, Guangzhou

梁煥枝師父

三久古勞詠春 廣州

Content

Foreword

The Tai Chi Classics is a collection of a hundred essays written by the most authoritative past masters on the subject of Tai Chi Chuan, largely intact and passed down through different lineages to the present day. Among those, the most famous and widely studied is the first essay in the collection, the 王宗岳太極拳論 Wang Zongyue Tai Chi Treatise. Supposedly discovered in a salt shop in Beijing during the mid-19th century, the Treatise is without a doubt one of the most important essays on the fundamentals of Tai Chi. It can be viewed as the essence of the entire collection, much like the Heart Sutra is the heart of the Diamond Sutra, and the Diamond Sutra is the heart of Buddhism. It is widely accepted that the Treatise was written by the martial arts scholar around the 13th to the 15th century.

The mechanics and methods described in the Treatise are universal and not unique to the discipline of Tai Chi. Its principles can be adapted in almost all areas of combat arts. To say that Wang Zongyue's treatise is relevant only to Tai Chi is as ludicrous as saying *Sun's Art of War* is applicable only to ancient warfare. It does not matter what styles of martial arts you do; the Wang Zongyue Tai Chi Treatise is a masterpiece that you will find useful time and again.

The central theme of the Wang Zongyue Tai Chi Treatise can be seen in paragraph three, 學力而有為, which means "achievement through studying force." He also advised practitioners not to 捨近求遠, to let go of the near to chase after the far.

Unfortunately, the Wang Zongyue Tai Chi Treatise is often misunderstood and sometimes even ridiculed by people who could not understand it. The Treatise is about the practical methods of manipulating and handling force; there is nothing esoteric or mystical, nor anything hidden in the text. The methods described are as relevant today as they were centuries ago. However, to understand the Treatise, one must see it through the eyes of a martial arts practitioner in a past culture vastly different from ours. This makes it impossible to interpret correctly without some diligent studies. Thus, some practitioners completely ignore this invaluable piece of writing, while others perceive it as a form of hidden alchemy.

I have spent close to forty years cultivating and refining my martial arts practice. The financial and personal costs I have invested in searching for the truth are incalculable. I have looked for masters from all over the world who could lead me on the right path. To them, especially my two Shifus, the late Imperial Yang Tai Chi Grandmaster Wei Shuren 魏樹人 and the late Sanjiu Kulo Wing Chun Master Leung Wunzi 梁煥枝, and the numerous teachers who had helped me along the way, I am eternally grateful.

One of the first things my teacher, Wei Shuren, went through with me when I got accepted into his discipleship is the dissection of the Tai Chi Classics. Out of all the essays, Grandmaster Wei placed the most importance on this Wang Zongyue Tai Chi Treatise. When Grandmaster Wei first went through it with me, there were many concepts I couldn't fully understand. However, he always advised me to write them down first, and over time, as my understanding deepens, I will be able to apply the written methods and fully appreciate his explanations. The key, he said, was to keep it simple and applicable. It took me a couple of decades to be proficient enough to comment on the Treatise in my own words. There are many beautifully translated versions of the Wang Zongyue Tai Chi Treatise in the public domain. With the poetic style of ancient Chinese writing, words can have multiple meanings and connotations. Every translator will inevitably incorporate their own interpretations into the translation; without subject-matter expertise, misinterpretation and incomplete translations are inevitable. Unless the translator understands, cultivates, and can apply the knowledge in practice, meanings are often lost or misrepresented.

This reference manual is a companion to my workshops on the Wang Zongyue Tai Chi Treatise, which I hold regularly in Australia and internationally. The first time I publicly ran the workshop was at the University of Technology, Sydney, around a decade ago. Since then, I have fine-tuned the workshops to become even more practical and easily understandable. I have kept this manual as concise and direct as possible. Those who have read my books and articles would know my style of writing; I am not going to waste my time and yours by padding this book with useless texts. I will keep things in a logical sequence and in a language that you should readily understand.

Everything described in the Wang Zongyue Tai Chi Treatise can be demonstrated at my workshops. There is nothing hidden in his writing. When you are willing to empty your cup and look at the Treatise with fresh eyes, you too will be able to carry out the methods written in these pages.

I hope you will find this manual useful on your martial arts journey.

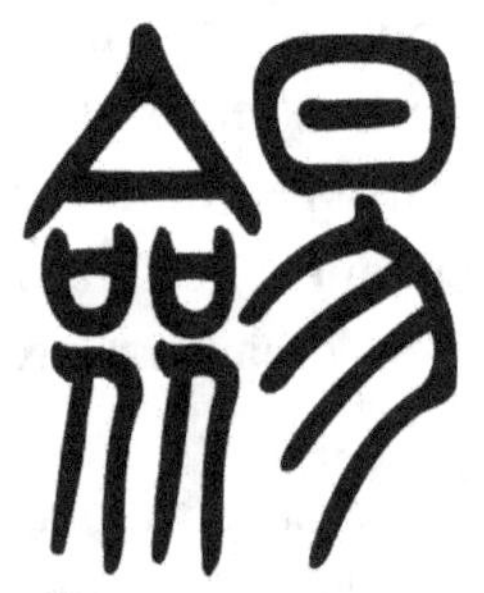

Dr. John K. Fung
www.MindBodyQi.com
November 2024

Original Text and Translation

The following pages contain the most widely used Chinese version of Wang Zongyue's Tai Chi Treatise, which I have then translated into English. You won't fully understand this translation until you go through it line by line in the following chapters. The numbers in brackets at the beginning of each line correlate to the numbers on the headings of the corresponding paragraphs, organised into chapters, for easy referencing. The translation may appear truncated, as I am trying to adhere to the original text as much as possible with minimal injection of personal views. Please study the expanded explanations to make sense of the texts and translations.

This manual is a supplement to my workshops. Feeling the concepts in person will help you understand and apply them faster.

王宗岳太極拳論

太極者，無極而生，（動靜之機，）陰陽之母也。動之則分，靜之則合。無過不及，隨曲就伸。人剛我柔謂之走，我順人背謂之黏。動急則急應，動緩則緩隨。雖變化萬端，而理唯一貫。由著熟而漸悟懂勁，由懂勁而階及神明，然非用力之久，不能豁然貫通焉。

虛領(靈)頂勁，氣沉丹田。不偏不倚，忽隱忽現。左重則左虛，右重則右杳。仰之則彌高，俯之則彌深。進之則愈長，退之則愈促。一羽不能加，蠅蟲不能落。人不知我，我獨知人。英雄所向無敵，蓋皆由此而及也。

斯技旁門甚多，雖勢有區別，概不外壯欺弱，慢讓快耳。有力打無力，手慢讓手快，是皆先天自然之能，非關學力而有為也。察「四兩撥千斤」之句，顯非力勝，觀耄耋能禦眾之形，快何能為。

立如枰準，活似車輪。偏沉則隨，雙重則滯。
每見數年純功，不能運化者，率皆自為人制，
雙重之病未悟耳。

欲避此病，須知陰陽。黏即是走，走即是黏。
陰不離陽，陽不離陰，陰陽相濟，方為懂勁。
懂勁後愈練愈精，默識揣摩，漸至從心所欲。

本是捨己從人，多誤捨近求遠，所謂「差之毫
釐，謬之千里」，學者不可不詳辨焉，是為
論。

Translation Overview

Wang Zongyue Tai Chi Treatise

(1) Taiji, born from Wuji, (the mechanics/moment of movement and stillness), mother of Yin and Yang. It separates upon movement, unites upon stillness. (2) No excess nor deficiencies; comfortably bends and casually extends. (3) When the other person is Gang and I am Rou, it is termed Zou; when I am fluid and the other person is awkward, it is termed Nian. (4) Quick movements require quick responses; slow movements require slow following. (5) Even though there are ten thousand variations, it is threaded by one principle. From familiarity to gradual understanding of Jin, from understanding Jin it touches divinity. Without manipulating force for a long time, there will be no breakthrough.

(6) Emptying the collar (agility) and Jing at the crown of the head; (7) Qi sinking to Dantian. (8) No slanting nor leaning, unpredictably hidden and appearing. (9) When the left is heavy, then left is emptied; when the right is heavy, then right disappears. (10) Looking up, it becomes higher; looking down, it becomes deeper. Advancing it becomes more distanced, retreating the more trapped. (11) A feather cannot add; a flying insect cannot land. (12) Others cannot read me; I alone read them. When a hero becomes invincible, it is all because of these.

(13) There are many side-door techniques; although the structures may differ, it is no more than the strong

bullying the weak, slow giving way to the fast. (14)
Strength overcomes weakness, slower hands give way to
faster hands; these are all natural abilities; it is not the
result of studying force. (15) Observe the phrase "four
taels displace a thousand catties," obviously it is not
winning by force. Watching a person in his/her eighties or
nineties manages to handle multiple opponents—how fast
can it be?

(16) Stand like a balancing scale (Cheng Zhun), (17)
mobile like a wheel (wheel-barge). (18) Polarised sinking
leads to fluidity; Double-Weightiness leads to stagnation.
(19) When you see someone with years of diligent
practice fails to practically apply his training and still
become controlled by others, it is because the sickness of
Double-Weightiness is not recognised yet.

(20) To remove this sickness, one must know Yin Yang.
(21) Nian is Zou, Zou is Nian. (22) Yin without leaving
Yang, Yang without leaving Yin, Yin and Yang nourish
each other; only then will you understand Jin. (23) Once
you know Jin, the more you practice, the more proficient
you become. Silently you explore; with time you can
perform whatever your heart desires.

(24) It is supposed to be letting go of self and flow with
others, but many mistakenly let go of the near to chase
after the far, as in the phrase "deviating by the least bit,
resulting in missing by a thousand miles." Practitioners
must not neglect the study. This is the Treatise.

Tai Chi Classics:
The Science of Manipulating Force
Workshop Outline

The following chart is the standard national and international workshop outline for the Wang Zongyue methods of manipulating force. Please use it as a guide only; we can customise it to meet the requirements of specific groups or schools. The methods are universal and can be adapted to almost all martial art styles.

Tai Chi Classics
Science of Manipulating Force
Workshop Outline

Understanding the Shen Yi Qi Command Chain	神為帥心為令氣為旗
	Theory
	Comet exercise
	Asking Star exercise
	Yin Yang 180 degree exchange exercise
	Asking Star Yin within Yin exercise
	High Pat Horse 180 degree ring exercise
Yin Yang Force Separation	動靜之機
	Theory: Refer to Wang Zongyue
	Location of Jinyuan
	Self listening
	Listening to partner
	Using Peng to displace opponent at Jinyuan
Adhering and Yielding	沾黏走化
	Theory: Refer to Wang Zongyue
	The 12 Yin Nails
	Silk Reeling: Self
	Silk Reeling: Opponent
	The 90 Degrees Rule
	The 3 gates
	Basic and Advanced Hand Circling Exercises
Combined Centre of Gravity CCoG	引進落空合即(極)出
	Theory: The 3 centres of gravity
	Theory: The power base
	Taking the partner off his power base
	Learning to listen to the CCoG
	Moving with the CCoG
	Destabilising the opponent with CCoG
Left-Right Energy Exchange	Refer to Wang Zongyue
	No slanting, sink the Qi
	Left-Right energy exchange drill
	Advanced: Up, down, enter, retreat

continue next page

Core Stability: Balancing Scale and Wheel	立如枰準，活似車輪
	Refer to Wang Zongyue
	Stability-Mobility continuum
	本固任從枝葉動 Stable trunk moving branches exercise
Back Aura W-Shaped Energy Exchange	背貼氣 山字訣
	Theory: Energy Structure
	Creating the Back Aura through Mingmen
	Yin within Yin, W-Shaped energetics
Polarised Sinking Double Weightiness	偏沉，雙重
	Theory: Refer to Wang Zongyue
	Recognising the Polarised Sinking
	Revisit the 90 degrees rule
	Opponent-Self Polarised Sinking
	Left-Right Polarised Sinking
	Top-Bottom Polarised Sinking
Advanced Yin Yang Principles	Wang Zongyue definition of Adhering and Yielding
	聽問拿放 Listen, Ask, Seize, Release
	Adhering=Yielding exercise
	Stability using Yin Yang opposition
	Power Manipulation through contact point
Advanced Method of Following the Opponent	Borrowing Yi Qi
	Workshop recap, no-mind

Paragraph I

太極者，無極而生，（動靜之機，）陰陽之母也。動之則分，靜之則合。無過不及，隨曲就伸。人剛我柔謂之走，我順人背謂之黏。動急則急應，動緩則緩隨。雖變化萬端，而理唯一貫。由著熟而漸悟懂勁，由懂勁而階及神明，然非用力之久，不能豁然貫通焉。

Taiji, born from Wuji, (the mechanics/moment of movement and stillness), mother of Yin and Yang. It separates upon movement, unites upon stillness. No excess nor deficiencies; comfortably bends and casually extends. When the other person is Gang and I am Rou it is termed Zou; when I am fluid and the other person is awkward, it is termed Nian. Quick movements require quick responses; slow movements require slow following. Even though there are ten thousand variations, it is threaded by one principle. From familiarity to gradual understanding of Jin, from understanding Jin it touches divinity. Without manipulating force for a long time, there will be no breakthrough.

The first paragraph of the Tai Chi Treatise outlines the overall mechanics of Taiji, the most important key points, and lays down the definitions of technical terms.

1. 太極者，無極而生，
（動靜之機，）陰陽之母也。
動之則分，靜之則合。

Translation:

Taiji, born from Wuji, (the mechanics/moment of movement and stillness), mother of Yin and Yang. It separates upon movement, unites upon stillness.

Explanation:

The opening statement summarises the nature of movement.

What Wang Zongyue was trying to establish is the universal law of movement. The Wuji state exists prior to movement. The Wuji state is undifferentiated. There are no opposing forces.

Before your opponent can move, he must first, for lack of a better word, "polarise" his body. This manifests the Taiji state, requiring the activation of his mind, consolidation of his body, differentiation of balance, initiation of movements, and generation of forces. Forces always come in pairs; the creation of one force vector (Yang) always results in the creation of an equal and opposite vector (Yin). The more the opponent presses against you, the stronger the opposing forces become; and the separation between Yin and Yang increases. Yin and Yang is the nature of all interactions. The generation of forces follow the sequence from Wuji to Taiji to Yin and Yang. This is a physical law; no one can get around this. As the conflict is

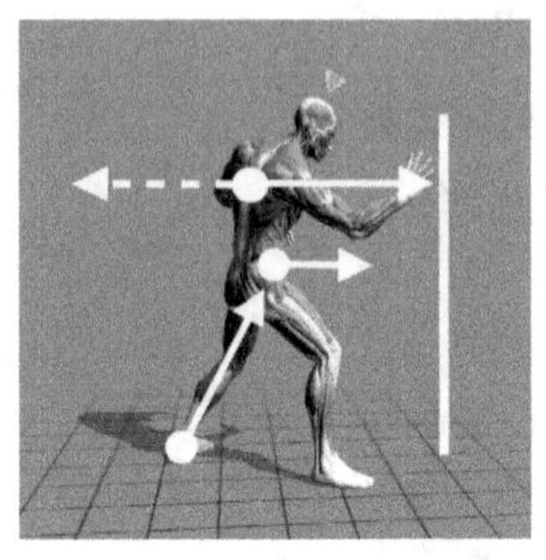

resolved, the Yin and Yang dissolve back into Wuji.

You can try this yourself: Find yourself an immovable object, then push against it. Observe that the more you attempt to exert forward force, the more it pushes back into you. If you are generating the force through your arms, the reflective point where the Yin Yang separation occurs will be at the 勁源 Jinyuan, Power Source, located between your shoulder blades. To compensate, you may need to move your centre of gravity forward. If you generate your force through different parts of your body, the location of the Jinyuan will change. However, there will always be a Yin Yang separation, and you will need to adjust your body to compensate for this. Please take your time to feel the changes in forces and structural alignment. This is only the first step.

When an opponent pushes against you, he must go through the same process that you have just experienced. By feeling the way your opponent tries to separate his Yin Yang, you can catch the formation of the Taiji state within the opponent and dominate the beginning of the separation and disable your opponent before he could generate any force. You will not have to fight force against force, and you will be able to defeat him with little effort.

If you can understand why Taiji is "the mechanics/ moment of movement and stillness, mother of Yin and

Yang" and see the rest of the essay in the light of practical mechanics, you will begin to make sense of the Wang Zongyue Tai Chi Treatise.

2. 無過不及，隨曲就伸。

Translation:

No excess nor deficiencies; comfortably bends and casually extends.

Explanations:

If one chooses to engage an opponent, there are essentially two ways to deal with his incoming force. You can either fight against it or you can work with it. In Wang Zongyue's model, you would opt to work with the force. Working with the force can be compared to jumping onto a moving bus. You must align yourself with the bus's movement; if you are too fast or too slow, excessive or insufficient, you will fall over. Similarly, to stay balanced while standing on the same bus, you must bend and extend your body comfortably. You are not moving according to your will but following along with the movement of the bus. You are working with the momentum, inertia, and balance.

Whether you are riding a bicycle, surfing the waves, riding a mechanical bull, or dealing with an opponent, it is the same. You do not fight the object; you work with it. Your actions are casual, and you need to remain comfortable. Balancing requires no conscious effort. By the time you think about how to balance, you will have already fallen off. If you fight the surfboard or the bicycle through deliberate or unnatural movements, you will fail.

Dealing with an opponent is no different. Obviously, if you are significantly stronger than your opponent physically, you can oppose him and dominate him with brute force. Otherwise, the best choice of action is to work with him, be it internally or externally, similar to the examples above.

3. 人剛我柔謂之走，
我順人背謂之黏。

Translation:

When the other person is Gang and I am Rou it is termed Zou; when I am fluid and the other person is awkward, it is termed Nian.

Explanations:

The most common translations of 黏 Nian and 走 Zou are Adhering and Yielding. There are numerous arguments within the Tai Chi and martial arts community regarding the meanings of these terms. However, Wang Zongyue had clearly defined these terms, so there's really no point in arguing over their meanings unless one doubts the authority of the author.

Wang Zongyue defined Zou, Yielding, as when the opponent is 剛 Gang, and you respond with 柔 Rou. But what is Gang, and what is Rou?

Like most Chinese words, Gang has multiple associated meanings. However, it all points towards something rigid and a quality of forcefulness. According to the 說文 Shuowen Dictionary, Gang is the sound when a knife hits metal, and Rou is "wood that can be bent and straightened." The pictogram of the word 柔 actually means "spear-wood 矛-木." Thus, Rou does not just mean soft. According to the 康熙 Kangxi Dictionary, Rou is the opposite of Gang. When attempting to understand the terms Gang and Rou, it is important to consider their underlying associated meanings, rather than simply focusing on the terms "hard" and "soft."

The term Zou states, "when the opponent is Gang and I am Rou." There is no ambiguity here, as the term is clearly defined.

Next, Wang Zongyue defined Nian, Adhering, as when you are 順 Shun and the opponent is 背 Bei.

順 Shun has the associated meaning of going along with something instead of against it, and it conveys a quality of comfort, casualness, and effortlessness. Conversely, 背 Bei is associated with going against, feeling of awkwardness and discomfort, and actions that require effort.

According to Wang Zongyue, if you are simply sticking to the opponent without making him feel Bei, you are not doing the Nian correctly. Only when you feel comfortable and your opponent feels awkward while adhering can you truly cultivate Nian.

In a later part of the Treatise there is another reference to Zou and Nian. We shall explore the concepts further in the later chapter.

4. 動急則急應，動緩則緩隨。

Translation:
Quick movements require quick responses; slow movements require slow following.

Explanations:
Many martial artists find this statement illogical. The argument is that it's always preferable to be faster than your opponent. Obviously, if you are striking the opponent or opposing him, the faster you are the better. However, when it comes to manipulating force, too fast or too slow will lead to conflict. The methods described by Wang Zongyue are about overcoming greater force by working with the force. Timing, therefore, must be just right.

This is not to say you would not want to finish the fight quickly. However, you can achieve this by timing your responses correctly, not by moving faster.

To move at the right pace, you must be able to follow the opponent, grasp the transition from Wuji to Taiji states, possess neither excess nor deficiencies, and correctly apply Zou and Nian, as previously described.

5. 雖變化萬端，而理唯一貫。
由著熟而漸悟懂勁，
由懂勁而階及神明，
然非用力之久，不能豁然貫通焉。

Translation:
Even though there are ten thousand variations, it is threaded by one principle. From familiarity to gradual understanding of Jin, from understanding Jin it touches divinity. Without manipulating force for a long time, there will be no breakthrough.

Explanations:
The underlying principle described by Wang Zongyue is universal. Different martial arts styles may have different variations in forms, but the underlying principles of clever force handling are always the same.

So what is Jin 勁?

It is not solely about power or force, as some may explain. Again, we may have a better grasp of the meaning by looking at the composition of the compound word:

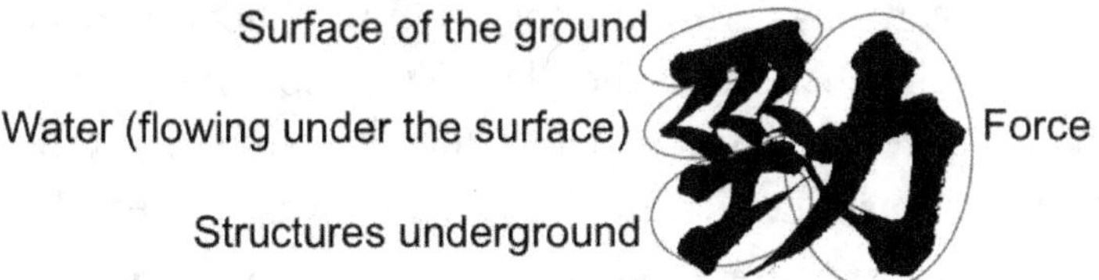

27

As illustrated on the previous page, Jin consists of four components: the surface of the ground, water flowing under the surface, structures underground, and force. Therefore, we can understand Jin as "forces that flow like water underground."

Wong Zongyue said that you will not have a thorough understanding of Jin unless you spend some time studying it. Beginners may find it hidden and difficult to experience. It's similar to balancing on a bicycle; you either know it or you don't. And similar to balancing on a bicycle, the breakthrough on the realisation of Jin is sudden. Of course, once you realise it, you will need to keep practicing and refining your skills.

Wang Zongyue described your skills as reaching "神明 Shen Ming," a term that can be loosely translated as "divinity" or "God-like." We can more accurately translate this term as "Shen Shining." The word for Shen 神 is made up of a picture of an altar 礻 on the left and a bolt of lightning 申 on the right. It has the connotation of spirituality and an all-powerful flash of connection between heaven and earth, like a bolt of lightning. Ming 明 is shining, like the Sun 日 and the Moon 月, which encompasses Yin and Yang and all things. Shen represents the instantaneous realisation that your true identity lies in the non-self. Shen heads the Shen-Yi-Qi command chain, which I have discussed in detail in my previous books, Practical Tensiometrics and Yi 意. It is a vast subject; I will not elaborate here. Shen Ming is the expression of the superconsciousness beyond your awareness that

encompasses all. When Wang Zongyue talked about Shen
Ming, it may be interpreted as the highest form of function
in many disciplines and arts. It has nothing to do with
deities.

Paragraph II

虛領(靈)頂勁，氣沉丹田。不偏不倚，忽隱忽現。左
重則左虛，右重則右杳。仰之則彌高，俯之則彌深。
進之則愈長，退之則愈促。一羽不能加，蠅蟲不能
落。人不知我，我獨知人。英雄所向無敵，蓋皆由此
而及也。

*Emptying the collar (agility) and Jing at the crown of the
head, Qi sinking to Dantian. No slanting nor leaning,
unpredictably hidden and appearing. When the left is
heavy, then left is emptied; when the right is heavy, then
right disappears. Looking up, it becomes higher; looking
down, it becomes deeper. Advancing it becomes more
distanced, retreating the more trapped. A feather cannot
add; a flying insect cannot land. Others cannot read me; I
alone read them. When a hero becomes invincible, it is all
because of these.*

The second paragraph of Wang Zongyue's Tai Chi Treatise
is mainly concerned with the static structures of force
handling.

6. 虛領(靈)頂勁

Translation:
Emptying the collar (agility) and Jing at the crown of the head.

Explanations:
There are a number of interpretations of this line, but fundamentally, they point towards the same results. Please bear with me, as this can get rather confusing and convoluted. However, I do not want to impose my personal preferred interpretation; I want you to understand the various words and arrive at your own conclusion.

1. 虛 Xu

虛 Xu implies insubstantial, no-force, weakness, and emptying of the content of a structure but not its physicality. It also has a connotation of deception. For example, a person with 氣虛 Qi Xu means there is a weakness in the person's Qi, although physically and structurally you may not see any signs. Another example, a 虛谷 Xu Gu is a ravine that appears to be empty, yet it remains physically present.

2. 領/靈 Ling

Although the pronunciation is the same, some sources refer to the word as 領, while others use the word 靈, and the implications can be quite different.

The first 領 Ling, referring to the collar, can also mean "leading." Therefore, Xu Ling can signify emptying the collar, implying that your neck should be upright and lightly touch your collar. It can also allude to the manipulation of power through "leading by the insubstantial."

The second 靈 Ling stands for spiritedness and agility. Thus Xu Ling, in this sense, could mean "lightness, spiritedness, and agility."

3. 頂 Ding

頂 Ding may refer to the crown of your head or the action of pushing upright.

4. 勁 Jin

勁 Jin I have explained it in Paragraph II, line (5), so I will not repeat it here. Therefore, the term "頂勁 Ding Jin" can refer to the act of pushing one's head upright or the state of being upright.

The most common interpretation of this line, Xu Ling Ding Jin 虛領(靈)頂勁, is "emptying the collar and pushing up the head." This line can also signify a combination of lightness, agility, and spiritedness, pushing upright and filled with Jin.

While the exact meanings are argued amongst scholars, the fundamental idea is that you must remain light, keeping your neck (thus the spine) erect, supported by your Jin.

7. 氣沉丹田

Translation:
Qi sinking to Dantian.

Explanations:
To explain the concept of Qi, it will take a whole book, if not more. I have elaborated on the subject in my previous books, *Practical Tensiometrics* and *Yi* 意; I will not go too deeply into it here.

While 氣 Qi is a hotly debated subject in Chinese martial arts, this is the only time Wong Zongyue mentioned it in his Treatise. It is crucial to understand that Qi does not refer to the air you breathe but rather to the sensation of an invisible "something" that you experience, although you can help feel it through breathing exercises.

Sinking your Qi is not pushing down your Qi. It is a natural settling process, like a pebble sinking in a pond. You don't need to exert any external force or effort. When sinking your Qi into the Dantian, you should feel comfortable and relaxed. Many people mistakenly believe that sinking the Qi involves physically lowering the body. The process occurs internally, concealing any visible movement. Similar to balancing on a bicycle, you can either balance or you can't. There is no visible difference between the person who can balance and someone who pretends to balance. You can lower your body as much as you like, but if you cannot sink the Qi, no amount of lowering will help you achieve it. Once you can sink the

Qi, you will gain a whole new level of stability and support.

Your 丹田 Dantian simply means "field of elixir." Depending on the martial art you study, there may be many Dantians in your body. In this Treatise, your Dantian is most likely referring to the general region of your lower abdomen and not the single Qihai 氣海 acupuncture point or multiple regions. If you can proficiently sink your Qi to the Dantian, you can do the same anywhere else in your body.

Note: Chinese poetry frequently employs opposites in its compositions. For example, Wang Zongyue thus far has used movements versus stillness, Yin versus Yang, Gang versus Rou, Shun versus Bei, and fast versus slow. Here, he used rising (of the crown) versus sinking (of the Qi). You can use this pattern to help decipher many old Chinese texts.

8. 不偏不倚，忽隱忽現。

Translation:

No slanting nor leaning, unpredictably hidden and appearing.

Explanation:

In Tai Chi, the ideas of "Central Stability, 中定 Zhong Ding" and "中正安舒 Centred, Upright, Peaceful, Comfortable, Zhong Zheng An Shu" are universal concepts. You may also see these ideas in other arts such as Wing Chun, Judo, and Aikido, where the practitioners remain balanced and upright while issuing power and performing their techniques.

Unless you are stronger than your opponent and he has no skills, you should never issue force by leaning into him. Once you shift your centre of gravity away from your base, you are providing your opponent with opportunities to manipulate you or disrupt your balance. You should be very mindful while pushing forward, as you may lose balance.

You shouldn't maintain your power continuously, as it makes it easy for your opponent to predict your attacks and defences, giving him an advantage over you. You should remain elusive so he cannot find you. Your power and movements should appear and disappear like a ghostly presence, leaving your opponent with nothing to work with. By the time your opponent senses your presence, he has already lost.

9. 左重則左虛，右重則右杳。

Translation:
When the left is heavy, then left is emptied; when the right is heavy, then right disappears.

Explanations:
It is common practice among the Tai Chi crowd to physically yield to an incoming force by moving away from it. However, this is not entirely correct, according to Wang Zongyue. The keyword here is Xu 虛, as in "when the left is heavy, the left becomes Xu." As previously mentioned, Xu means emptying a structure's content but not its appearance.

In 李亦畬 Li Yishe's Treatise, "左重則左虛，而右已去 when the left is heavy, the left becomes light, and power exits through the right."

Left and right are relative; they can be anywhere in the body. The return path can be any size; a highly skilled practitioner can return within a contact point.

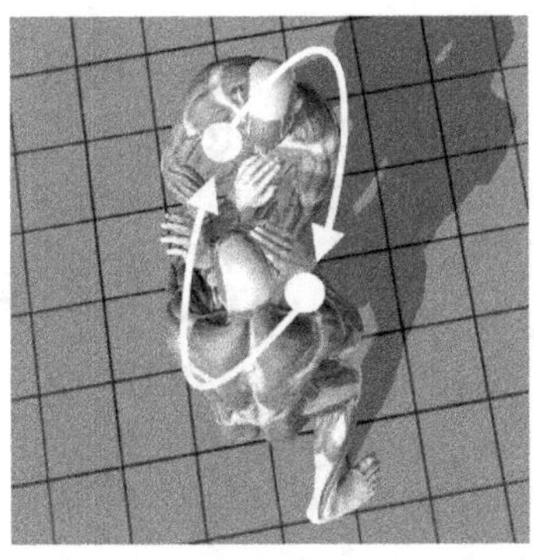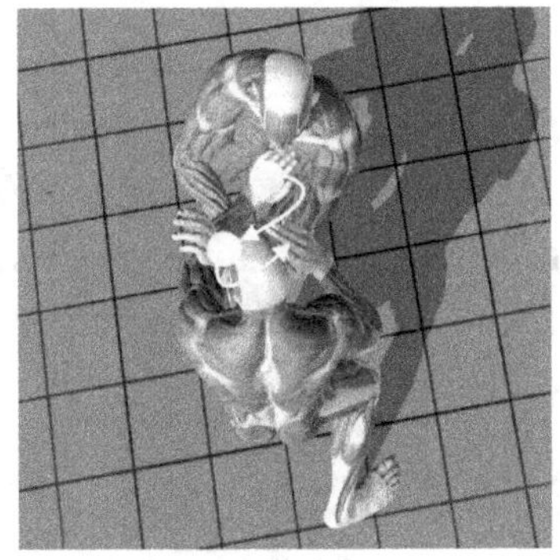

When an opponent is exerting a force on you, whether you feel the heaviness on the left or the right, you would need to empty it or make it disappear without perceivable physical movements. If you retreat, the opponent will pursue you, or he may modify his tactics to counter your counterattacks. Sooner or later, you will run out of options. By emptying with the least physical movement, you are deceiving your opponent, making it harder for him to retaliate. Wars are often won through deception. No one can fight what he cannot perceive.

Another misconception is that one can empty the opponent's force just by relaxing or being soft alone. He will continue to intensify his attack until you collapse. You cannot empty his force by absorbing it; you must drain it away somewhere. If you move the force to another part of the body, such as your feet, as taught by many martial arts teachers, your feet will become heavy, and you will not be able to empty it further, and it will be stuck there. If you are physically stronger than your opponent, that is not a problem; you can defeat him with brute force. If you have to overcome someone stronger than you and your feet are stuck, it is not going to work.

The key, therefore, is to drain the force away, preferably back into your opponent through an alternate circuit, instead of just absorbing it. Wang Zongyue suggests using combinations of Gang and Rou, Zou and Nian, and Shun and Bei to drain the opponent's power back into him.

10. 仰之則彌高，俯之則彌深。
進之則愈長，退之則愈促。

Translation:

Looking up, it becomes higher; looking down, it becomes deeper. Advancing it becomes more distanced, retreating the more trapped.

Explanations:

The previous statements concern merely the emptying; here it takes one step further to create the illusion of the void.

Regardless of whether the opponent is directing his force upward, downward, or forward, you can create an illusion that makes him feel as though he is falling into a void. Again, this is not done by physical movements, because if he can perceive your intentions, he will not be deceived. This is done by subtly changing his balance by manipulating the Combined Centre of Gravity (CCoG) and returning the power to him where he is not aware of it. Your mind and body combine to create this illusion. When you train well, your body will obey your thoughts and behave accordingly. This is how the Shen-Yi-Qi command chain works. There is nothing mystical about it; it is neural science. One time, when I was training with late grandmaster Wei, he was issuing an 按 An, Push Down, energy on me. I could feel I was standing upright; his hands were light, but there was so much power going through me I had no choice but to fall down. Later, when my student showed me the video, I found myself leaning backwards and struggling to maintain my balance, which ultimately led to my fall. What I realised was that what Grandmaster Wei did was not some secret Qi blast technique; he fooled my senses in such a way that my body was defeating itself. You must avoid micromanaging your body to shift or soften using specific techniques, as any deliberate actions could reveal your intentions to the opponent, leaving you vulnerable to their counterattacks. To create this illusion, you have to do it without conscious thoughts, much like balancing on your bike while riding down a rocky path.

Trapping the opponent while he is retrieving requires more skills. When done properly, you are not grabbing him, yet he cannot escape, as if he is glued to you. This requires diligent practice and your cultivation of Nailing, Threading, and Freezing.

I have written extensively about the CCoG, Nailing, Threading, Freezing, and the Shen-Yi-Qi command chain in my previous books. There is not enough room to discuss these vast subjects here. Please refer to my previous publications.

11. 一羽不能加，蠅蟲不能落。

Translation:
A feather cannot add; a flying insect cannot land.

Explanations:
When you are interacting with your opponent, obviously there will be forces involved. However, you, not your opponent, set the limits on the amount of force allowed in the interaction. For instance, if you decide to allow four kilogrammes of force at the point of contact where you and your opponent meet, he will not be able to add more. A feather cannot add; it does not mean you have to be light as a feather; it means the weight of a feather cannot be added to what is already there.

Wong Zhongyue described the opponent as not being able to land their power onto us; figuratively speaking not even a flying insect can land.

If you train according to the methods set out in the Wang Zongyue Tai Chi Treatise, you will be able to achieve the effect that a feather cannot add and a flying insect cannot land. However, people often treat Tai Chi Push-Hand competitions as a form of sport wrestling, complete with their own set of rules and weight divisions. If your goal is to compete, you will need to train according to the quickest path to win your prize. Depending on the purpose of your training, these methods may or may not suit.

12. 人不知我，我獨知人。
英雄所向無敵，蓋皆由此而及也。

Translation:

Others cannot read me; I alone read them. When a hero becomes invincible, it is all because of these.

Explanations:

"All warfare is based on deceptions."
The Art of War, Sun Tzu

According to Wang Zhongyue, defeating your opponents requires deception. You are invincible if you can read your opponents, but they can't read you.

It does not matter what discipline you practice, from Tai Chi to Wing Chun, from other forms of combat arts to competitive sports such as tennis, and to corporate takeovers and international trade; the principle of knowing your opponent and hiding your intentions, resources, and strategies is universal.

Your Listening skill is of utmost importance. If you are not familiar with Tai Chi, Listening skill, or Ting Jin 聽勁, is your ability to sense the opponent's force and other vital information. Its function is similar to spies gathering intelligence about the enemy. If your opponent can deceive you, you will be defeated. But if you can sense and assess your opponent's intent and forces correctly, you can counter his every move.

47

One of the reasons why Wong Zhongyue did not advocate fighting force against force is related to deception. When your force is not hidden, your opponent will detect it and counter your techniques. As previously described, if you issue Jin, a hidden force, your opponent cannot fight against what he cannot perceive.

Paragraph III

斯技旁門甚多，雖勢有區別，概不外壯欺弱，慢讓快
耳。有力打無力，手慢讓手快，是皆先天自然之能，
非關學力而有為也。察「四兩撥千斤」之句，顯非力
勝，觀耄耋能禦眾之形，快何能為。

*There are many side-door techniques; although the
structures may differ, it is no more than the strong bullying
the weak, slow giving way to the fast. Strength overcomes
weakness, slower hands give way to faster hands; these
are all natural abilities; it is not the result of studying
force. Observe the phrase "four taels displace a thousand
catties," obviously it is not winning by force. Watching a
person in his/her eighties or nineties manages to handle
multiple opponents—how fast can it be?*

In this paragraph, Wong Zhongyue outlined what he
considered natural or athletic abilities developed through
physical techniques, which he described as side-door, and
what he considered "learning about force."

13. 斯技旁門甚多，雖勢有區別，
概不外壯欺弱，慢讓快耳。

Translation:

There are many side-door techniques; although the structures may differ, it is no more than the strong bullying the weak, slow giving way to the fast.

Explanations:

In my opinion, there is nothing wrong with being faster and stronger than your opponent.

However, Wang Zhongyue had observed that most martial arts styles are based on being faster and stronger than your opponents. He called these methods "side doors" and not the methods he described in his Treatise.

14. 有力打無力，手慢讓手快，
是皆先天自然之能，非關學力而有為也。

Translation:

Strength overcomes weakness, slower hands give way to faster hands; these are all natural abilities; it is not the result of studying force.

Explanations:

Wong Zongyue called being stronger and faster than your opponent "natural abilities." However, Tai Chi is about "學力," which means "studying force." Studying force is the central theme of his Treatise.

Notice that Wang Zongyue did not mention anything mystical about the practice of Tai Chi; he was completely pragmatic in his approach. He advocates learning about the nature of force and how to manipulate it instead of pursuing unrealistic goals, which may or may not be attainable.

Wong Zongyue did not forbid the use of force or speed; he merely said that it is a natural ability and has nothing to do with studying force.

15. 察「四兩撥千斤」之句，顯非力勝，
　　觀耄耋能禦眾之形，快何能為。

Translation:
Observe the phrase "four taels displace a thousand catties," obviously it is not winning by force. Watching a person in his/her eighties or nineties manages to handle multiple opponents—how fast can it be?

Explanations:
The proverb "Four taels displace a thousand catties" has become a cliché in Tai Chi practices. But how do we achieve this? One cannot simply wish for it to happen or believe that repeated practice alone can achieve it. In addition to diligent studies, one must understand and apply the mechanics.

Generally, the methods of moving the opponent with minimal force fall into three categories:

1. **Levers:** This is pretty obvious; the longer the lever, the higher the torque. This works both ways. For example, if an opponent applies a force to a point, such as grabbing our wrist, instead of fighting against his grab, keep the point as the centre of a circle, then move along the path of an arc, which is part of the circumference. The larger the radius, the less force is required to move the opponent or break the grip. This is the core principle of 移位不移點, moving the position without moving the point (of contact). Another example is that if your opponent tries to

move you, invite them to become overextended. The more he extends, the more difficult it becomes for him to generate his force.

2. **Balance:** Human beings stand and fight on two feet. This is an unstable equilibrium that requires constant automatic adjustment to remain upright. If you can deceive your opponent's senses, either by creating the illusion that he can lean on you and then abruptly removing it, or by luring him away from his power base, he will lose his balance. If he cannot balance, he cannot generate power.

3. **Stealth:** If you are sensitive enough, you will always find paths where there is minimal resistance. Find those paths, and you can drop your opponent with minimal force. He cannot resist what he cannot evaluate correctly.

4. **Pain and fear:** The opponent will naturally want to avoid situations that will cause them pain or anything that they fear. For instance, a joint lock could result in pain, while an attack on his face could evoke fear. The opponent's body will subconsciously move to avoid these, causing his structure to become compromised. He won't be able to generate power effectively if his structure is broken.

When you practice these techniques with a compliant partner, it is simple. However, a skilled opponent will not readily give away his weaknesses; therefore, you must play with his senses and his mind to achieve these results.

In terms of speed, if you are trying to manipulate his force, you do not need to move fast, but you would need

to adapt quickly. You do not need to be physically faster
than him, but you must adapt faster than him. When you
need to move quickly, for example, to block an incoming
strike, you must refine your techniques to become more
efficient and require less movement. Therefore, you will
be faster than him even though you are physically slower.

Paragraph IV

立如枰準，活似車輪。偏沉則隨，雙重則滯。每見數年純功，不能運化者，率皆自為人制，雙重之病未悟耳。

Stand like a balancing scale (Cheng Zhun), mobile like a wheel (wheel-barge). Polarised sinking leads to fluidity; Double-Weightiness leads to stagnation. When you see someone with years of diligent practice fails to practically apply his training and still become controlled by others, it is because the sickness of Double-Weightiness is not recognised yet.

Paragraph IV describes the importance of balance and fluidity and the problem of Double-Weightiness that many practitioners face.

16. 立如枰準

Translation:

Stand like a balancing scale (Cheng Zhun).

Explanations:

The most widely accepted translation of a 枰準 Cheng Zhun, refers to a balancing scale that one uses to weigh items. However, although the imagery accurately depicts a person standing upright and balanced, the balancing scale most people are familiar with is a Western instrument that was not widely used in China during Wang Zongyue's time.

Some practitioners interpret the Cheng Zhun as the 桿秤 Gan Cheng, pictured on the right. The Gan Cheng is operated by suspending it by a string; the counterweight is then moved along the rod to balance against 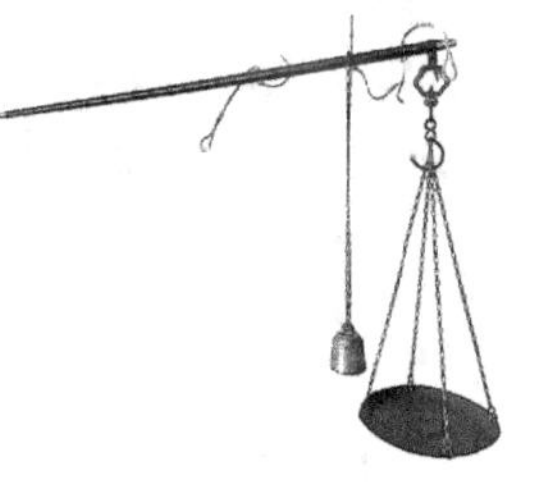 the item to be weighed on the tray. This adds to the element that, while the structures may look asymmetrical, the system as a whole is balanced and suspended, as in (6), "Emptying the collar (agility) and Jing at the crown of the head."

Another explanation suggested by some scholars is that the Cheng Zhun refers to an instrument described in various military texts as 平準 Ping Zhun. The writing is very similar. This is a sophisticated instrument with three

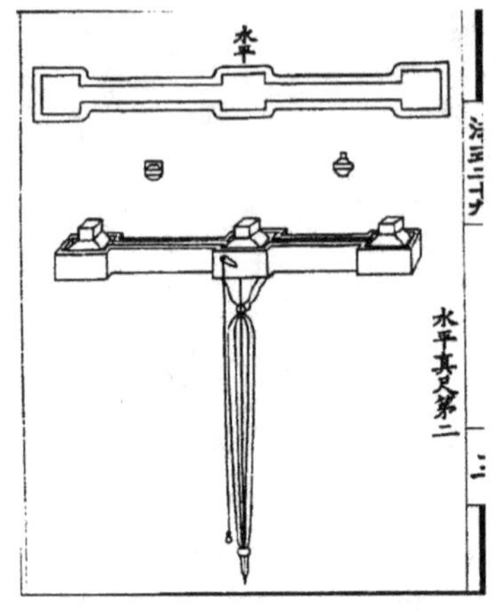

wooden blocks floating on water on the horizontal beam and a plumb-bob hanging down the middle. With this model, you would maintain internally levelled like water. In the 汪魏 Wang (Yongquan)-Wei (Shuren) Tai Chi lineage, we also incorporate an imaginary pendulum that is suspended from a referencing cross located in the chest.

Personally, I favour the Ping Zhun model; however, these are just anecdotes. As long as you are standing upright and balanced, you are adhering to the phrase 立如枰準.

17. 活似車輪

Translation:

Mobile like a wheel (wheel-boat).

Explanations:

Once you have established the 中定 Zhong Ding, or central equilibrium, the forces acting on you can be dissipated and returned back to the opponent like a spinning wheel, as described by 李亦畬 Li Yishe. 左重則左虛，而右已去, when the left is heavy, the left becomes light and power exits through the right. Please refer to sentence (9) in Paragraph II. Similar to a wheel, this force returns passively, revolving in response to the applied force. The axis of rotation initially corresponds to your axis of balance, but as you improve, it can be anywhere in your body or outside.

An alternate interpretation of 車輪 wheel is the 車輪舸, or the wheel-barge.

The wheel-barge is a vessel used by the navy during the Ming Dynasty and around the time of Wang Zongyue. A pair of wheels on both sides propel the wheel-barge,

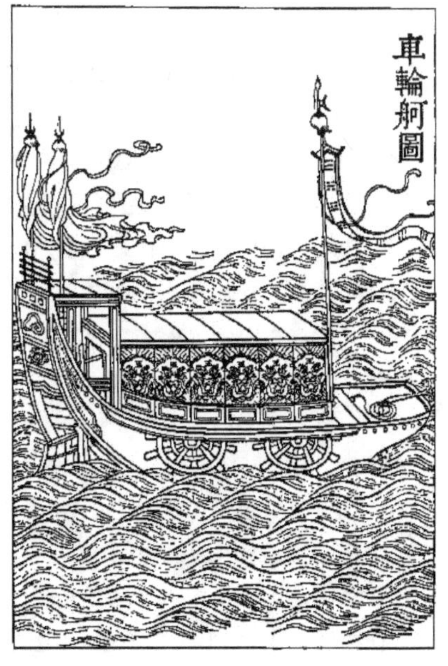

enabling it to manoeuvre 360 degrees while maintaining its upright and stable position. According to the traditional structure of Chinese poetry, if Wong Zhongyue referred his previous sentence to military equipment, it is likely that he would refer 車輪 to a navy vessel as well. This interpretation also adds to the dimension of mobility while remaining upright and stable. Thus the two sentences of (6)(7) "Emptying the collar (agility) and Jing at the crown of the head, Qi sinking to Dantian" juxtapose against the sentences (16)(17) "Stand like a balancing scale (Cheng Zhun), mobile like a wheel (wheel-boat)."

There are two ways to be mobile like a wheel: 1. by physically moving and rotating like a wheel, or 2. by not moving but transmitting the power back to the opponent without perceptible movement. The first method can be easily observed and learned; however, by the very nature that it can be easily observed, it can be easily sensed and countered by the opponent. The second method is done with hidden Jin. It is more effective because the opponent or observer cannot counter what he cannot easily perceive. Unfortunately, this method's inherent hiddenness makes it challenging to learn through books or even videos. However, if you experience it firsthand in one of my workshops, you will find it to be quite simple to implement.

Again, the various interpretations are simply anecdotes; I am providing these alternative perspectives for your contemplation. As long as you are moving freely and returning the power to the opponent, you can follow whatever interpretations align with your training.

18. 偏沉則隨，雙重則滯。

Translation:
Polarised sinking leads to fluidity; Double-Weightiness leads to stagnation.

Explanation:
These two sentences are crucial when dealing with non-compliant opponents.

What is 雙重 Double-Weightiness? This is a scientific concept. Just like two conductors with similar electrical charges, or two objects of similar temperatures, or two opponents issuing force with similar strengths, or both feet equally weighted, or the stability-mobility dynamic with undifferentiated lightness and heaviness. Basically, any system with a similar amount of Yang'ness or Yin'ness has a slow and stagnant transfer of energy. These are all forms of 雙重 Double-Weightiness.

When two opponents engage each other, they in effect become one closed system. When they are opposing each other, there is mutual struggle. To flow freely, there must be a potential difference between the relative Yin and the relative Yang. Wang Zongyue referred to this as 偏沉, polarised sinking. Therefore, when the opponent is heavy, we become light. When the opponent tries to be light, we sink him down. When there is a point of stillness, we counter it with mobility. We sink one side of the body and let the other side move freely. To remain stable, our base should be heavy while the top becomes light. We can generate power either by having a stable base and an agile upper body or by being light on our feet but with heavy arms.

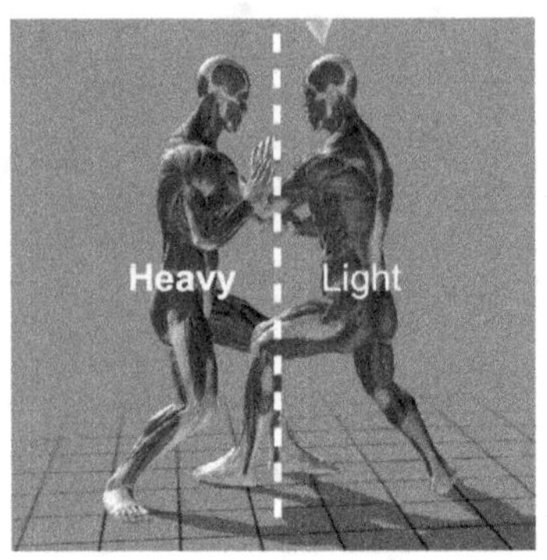

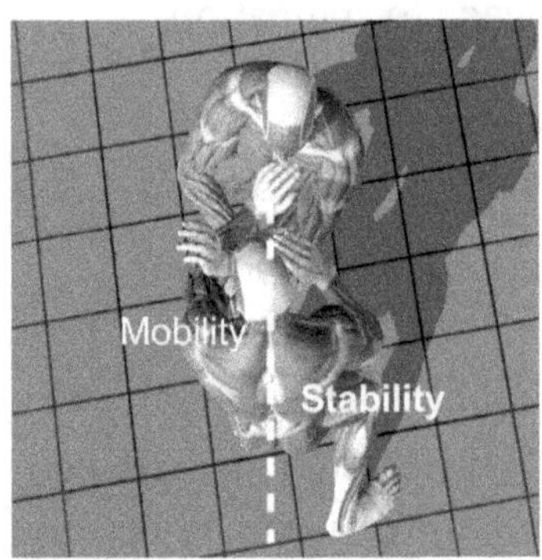

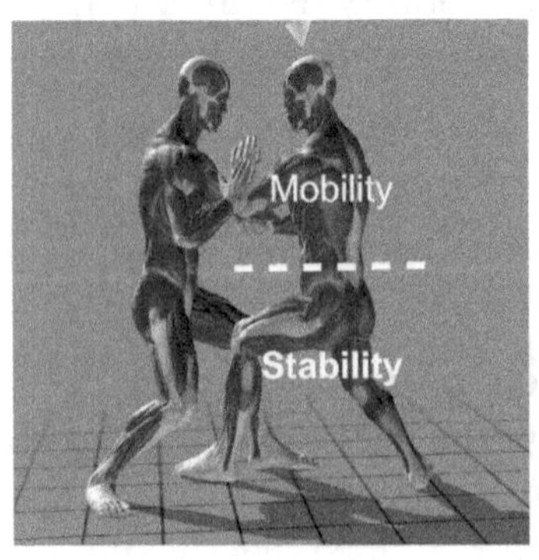

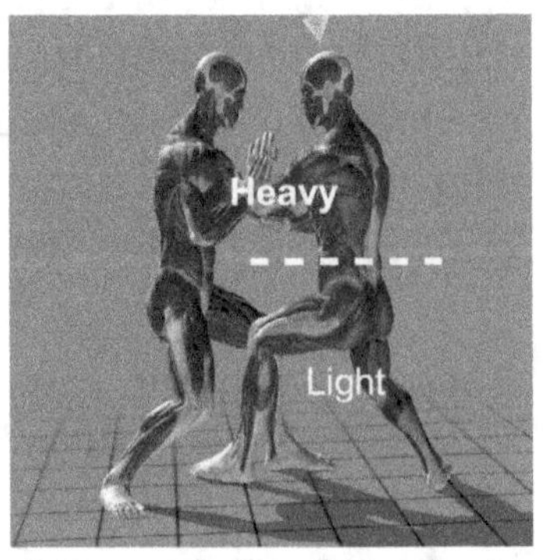

The 雙重 and 偏沉 are not absolute but relative. The relativity of the two concepts will be discussed later in the paragraph.

19. 每見數年純功，不能運化者，
率皆自為人制，雙重之病未悟耳。

Translation:

When you see someone with years of diligent practice fails to practically apply his training and still become controlled by others, it is because the sickness of Double-Weightiness is not recognised yet.

Explanations:

Clearly, the stronger prevails when strength meets strength. This paragraph demonstrates the practicality of Wang Zongyue's Tai Chi Treatise, as he not only explained the strategies, science, and structural requirements, but also provided advice on why people fail despite years of practice. He identified Double-Weightiness as the primary cause of failure. Time and time again, I see practitioners with supposedly years of experience resorting back to using brute force because of this. If your opponent's strength surpasses yours due to factors such as size, age, or athletic ability, you will ultimately lose.

Many of us are not even aware of the sickness of Double-Weightiness.

Paragraph V

欲避此病，須知陰陽。黏即是走，走即是黏。陰不離陽，陽不離陰，陰陽相濟，方為懂勁。懂勁後愈練愈精，默識揣摩，漸至從心所欲。

To remove this sickness, one must know Yin Yang. Nian is Zou, Zou is Nian. Yin without leaving Yang, Yang without leaving Yin, Yin and Yang nourish each other; only then will you understand Jin. Once you know Jin, the more you practice, the more proficient you become. Silently you explore; with time you can perform whatever your heart desires.

Paragraph V explains how to overcome the sickness of Double-Weightiness.

20. 欲避此病，須知陰陽。

Translation:
To remove this sickness, one must know Yin Yang.

Explanations:
To avoid Double-Weightiness, embrace Yin Yang. As mentioned before, flow occurs between Yin and Yang, from high potentials to low potentials. If neither you nor your opponent is exerting any force, there is no flow; this is the ideal situation because it signifies peace, as no one is actively opposing the other. If both of you use force, stagnation occurs, and the stronger person wins. Therefore, to handle an opponent the Wang Zongyue way, you should respond with suppleness when your opponent issues force, as this will prevent Double-Weightiness from occurring.

To gain a deeper understanding of the concept of avoiding Double-Weightiness, it is crucial to realise that Yin and Yang are not absolute but rather relative in terms of quality, time, and space.

For instance, Double-Weightiness occurs when both you and your opponent are similarly soft or hard. However, if your opponent is soft and you are softer, then Yin Yang is still present. When you and your opponent are both hard, as long as one of you is less hard, there exists Yin and Yang. While suppleness is supposed to defeat rigidity, it requires skills; if your opponent is less skilled and you have more strength, it is tempting to overpower him with strength. When we see people try to bulldoze each other with brute force, they are trying to defeat each other with strength instead of skills.

Double-Weightiness may also refer to time. Time Yin Yang pertains to variations in either speed or sequence. If both you and your opponent are opposing each other with similar speed, stagnation will occur. Fast will defeat slow, but this is athletic ability according to sentence (14); it has nothing to do with studying force. You may choose to slow down relative to your opponent and handle him with better efficiency instead of beating him by moving faster. This is described in sentence (15). Double-Weightiness may occur through sequence; according to sentence (8), your state of Yin and Yang should suddenly appear and disappear. You may meet your opponent with less power, then increase the output suddenly at the correct moment. You must not remain the same all the way through.

To avoid spatial Double-Weightiness, you must separate Yin and Yang through space. Instead of seeing you and your opponent as separate struggling systems, perceive the two of you as two regions within a closed system. To have flow, then one region must be relatively Yin, while the other becomes relatively Yang, or vice versa. You must determine who is Gang and who is Rou in relation to each other. When you see you and your opponent combined to form one system instead of two struggling systems with separate centres of gravity, namely your opponent's and yours, the system combines to form one single combined centre of gravity (CCoG). The CCoG flows naturally according to where the Yin and Yang are located within the system. Unless the opponent is well trained, he will not be able to detect the changes in the flow of the CCoG. Learning to manipulate the CCoG is an excellent way to control a Unified (合 He) system, thus the opponent indirectly. Once you are done with him, you can choose when to Separate (開 Kai) to repel him or to bounce him off. The topic of CCoG is extensive, so I won't delve into it further here. Please refer to my book *Practical Tensiometrics*.

My teacher, the late grandmaster Wei Shuren, advocated for the 49-51 rule, which states that when engaging an opponent, the separation of Yin and Yang should not have a large differentiation but rather a difference of 49 percent to 51 percent. This is because a skilled opponent can easily detect and counter a larger differentiation. At 49-51, it becomes elusive because to him, the difference is small. You may believe that the difference between 49 and 51 is insignificant, which is indeed true when viewed in its entirety. However, when viewed as a ratio of -1 to +1, the difference becomes significant. Grandmaster Wei always used to say, "You can defeat an opponent with the power of a grain of rice." That is, the small grains of -1 and +1.

I will explain more about Yin Yang later in this chapter.

21. 黏即是走，走即是黏。

Translation:
Nian is Zou, Zou is Nian.

Explanations:
This is the second point Wang Zongyue made regarding the method for removing the sickness of Double-Weightiness.

In Paragraph I sentence (3), Wang Zongyue defined Adhering (黏 Nian) and Yielding (走 Zou) as "when the other person is Gang and I am Rou, it is termed Zou; when I am fluid and the other person is awkward, it is termed Nian. 人剛我柔謂之走，我順人背謂之黏。" There is no need to argue over the meaning of these terms further unless you doubt the authority of Wang Zongyue.

We often see Tai Chi practitioners deal with the incoming force by adhering to the opponent and yielding, then pushing back with Gang power afterwards. While this strategy can be effective (refer to sentence (20) for the discussion of Time Yin Yang), it can result in Double-Weightiness if the opponent's force is not adequately dissipated or if one has taken too long to yield adequately and the opponent is given enough time to react and regains his power for subsequent attacks. In both of these scenarios, any attempts to push back will be met with a resisting force from the opponent, and once again the system becomes the Double-Weightiness of force against force.

When you yield only for the sake of yielding, it is Yin without Yang. Your opponent can comfortably continue to generate power. When you push back, you are being Gang, and you are no longer Rou.

According to Wang Zongyue, to eliminate Double-Weightiness, Nian is Zou, and Zou is Nian. Please refer back to the definitions of Zou (Yielding) and Nian (Adhering), Gang and Rou, Shun and Bei in Paragraph I statement (3).

According to this statement, when you apply Rou to the opponent's Gang, your suppleness against his strength, you must make him feel Bei, or stagnated, simultaneously. You must not respond to him with force, and at the same time you must not let him have the ability to generate force or move comfortably. If you respond to your opponent with Rou without stagnating him, he will be able to change and continue his attack on you. At a certain point in space and in time, you will reach a limit where you can no longer dissolve his attack. Once that point is reached, you will have to match him with force, thereby re-engaging the sickness of Double-Weightiness.

When we see practitioners requiring themselves to brace up for strong, wide stances to deal with their opponents, they are actually engaging Double-Weightiness no matter how much they claim they are adhering to the principles Adhering and Yielding. If they are truly being Rou, why would they need a strong, rigid stance? When you see Judo master Kyuzo Mifune throwing around other

Judokas twice his size, he never needed to brace up or get into strong stance. He remained light on his feet. We don't have videos of Wang Zongyue, but we have plenty of old videos of Mifune for you to contemplate.

The whole Treatise, up to this point, is about how to achieve Nian is Zou and Zou is Nian. Your opponent is supposed to lose his balance and his ability to generate power as soon as he engages with you. Sentence (11), which states that a feather cannot add and a fly cannot land, explains the effect of this. All the other parts of the Treatise describe how to achieve it.

22. 陰不離陽，陽不離陰，
陰陽相濟，方為懂勁。

Translation:

Yin without leaving Yang, Yang without leaving Yin, Yin and Yang nourish each other; only then will you understand Jin.

Explanations:

In the explanations for sentences (18) and (20), we have explored the necessities for polarised sinking and the fact that Yin and Yang are not absolutes but relative. Yin and Yang represent the inherent state of all things; it is impossible to have Yin without Yang, nor can Yang exist without Yin. Yin and Yang, by nature, support and nourish each other.

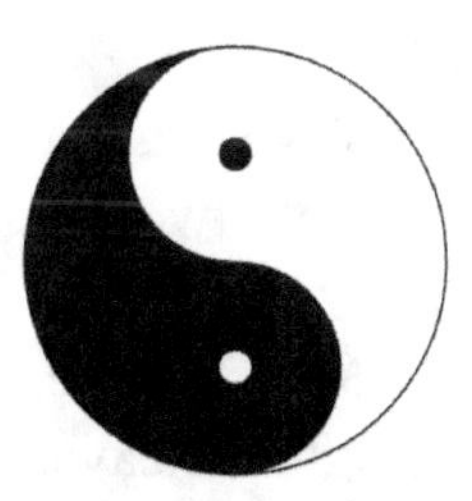

Yin and Yang can be found everywhere, but you will need to know where to look. If you look at the Taiji symbol, there is a black dot within the white and a white dot within the black. No matter how you want to separate Yin and Yang, there will always be a bit of the opposite within. For example, even in a Double-Weightiness system, when the opponent issues a Gang force against you, there will always be an equal and opposite force acting on him. If you can identify the specific part of his body, such as his Jinyuan or back leg, where the opposing force is acting, there you will find his black dot within the white. You can immediately convert the Double-Weightiness system into a Polarised Sinking system. When we discussed Grandmaster Wei's 49-51 method, it perfectly embodied the concept of the power of a grain of rice. Within the opponent's strength, there will also be a true weakness; within your Rou, there will always be a true Gang. This is how you will perform the methods described in (10), Looking up, it becomes higher; looking down, it becomes deeper. Advancing, it becomes more distanced, retreating the more trapped. From a third-person perspective, it would look like it is Double-Weightiness, that you are resisting, because there are no visual cues to suggest you are removing the opponent's force. Yet you are relaxed, Rou, and the opponent would feel either he is falling into a void or pushing against a mountain.

You can also think of Yin and Yang as having the same properties as fractals. They are infinitely divisible. When the opponent presses against your chest with a single palm, it may initially appear as if there is no Yin Yang. However, once you divide his area of contact into two halves, Yin and Yang re-establish themselves, allowing you to deal with him using the principles of (9): when the left is heavy, the left empties, and when the right is heavy, the right vanishes. You may return the power to him through the principle of (17), mobile like a wheel, within that single area of contact. When top-level masters send an opponent out with two fingers, they are essentially splitting the Yin and Yang along the index and middle fingers, thereby defeating the opponent through the use of a miniaturised Polarised Sinking.

You will easily topple over if your body is rigid. This is why people often practice having a low and wide stance while trying to keep the waist and arms mobile. To establish balance and stability, if you understand the principles of Yin and Yang, you will no longer need to brace up for such stances. From the Yin and Yang perspective, as long as the bottom half of the body is more stable than the top half, or the core is more stable than the periphery, you will become unmovable. As Yin and Yang are relative, as long as the contact point where the opponent is issuing his force is more unstable relative to your stance or your core, you will achieve stability. This implies that even if you are standing solely on one foot, as long as the contact points are less stable than your foot, your roots are still immovable and you will appear as a willow tree.

When you reach the level where you can redirect your opponent's power like the wheel without moving, as discussed in sentence (17), you will appear as solid as a stone tablet from a third person's perspective, yet you are remaining relatively Rou. 6th generation Chen style grandmaster 陳長興 Chen Changxing was nicknamed "Mr. Tablet" for his ability to do exactly this.

You won't understand Jin unless you can grasp these.

23. 懂勁後愈練愈精，默識揣摩，
漸至從心所欲。

Translation:
Once you know Jin, the more you practice, the more proficient you become. Silently you explore; with time you can perform whatever your heart desires.

Explanations:
Obviously, as with everything in life, the more you practice, the more proficiency you will achieve. The key statement here is 從心所欲, whatever your heart desires.

Again, we can use riding a bicycle as an example: In the beginning, you would pay a lot of attention to maintaining balance, but you would still fall over. However, once you have practiced enough, you can race down a rocky path without conscious effort. You still have to focus, but you no longer need to think. You ride as your heart desires.

Dealing with an opponent is exactly the same. Once you have practiced the methods written by Wang Zongyue and those presented in my workshops, you will eventually be able to deal with the opponent's force instinctively. You will still need to focus, but there is no conscious effort involved. This is the state of 無意出真意, where the true mind emerges from no mind. Whatever your heart desires, it is achieved.

Paragraph VI

本是捨己從人，多誤捨近求遠，所謂「差之毫釐，謬之千里」，學者不可不詳辨焉，是為論。

It is supposed to be letting go of self and flow with others, but many mistakenly let go of the near to chase after the far, as in the phrase "deviating by the least bit, resulting in missing by a thousand miles." Practitioners must not neglect the study. This is the Treatise.

This is the conclusion to the Wang Zongyue Tai Chi Treatise, and his final advice.

24. 本是捨己從人，多誤捨近求遠，
所謂「差之毫釐，謬之千里」，
學者不可不詳辨焉，
是為論。

Translations:

It is supposed to be letting go of self and flow with others, but many mistakenly let go of the near to chase after the far, as in the phrase "deviating by the least bit, resulting in missing by a thousand miles." Practitioners must not neglect the study. This is the Treatise.

Explanations:

I hope you can see by now that the Wang Zongyue Tai Chi Treatise is pragmatic and relatively easy to understand if you know how to look at it. Obviously, you will need to study this manual deeply and hopefully be able to attend my workshops to fully grasp the content. Once you have internalised all the methods, you will no longer need to make conscious efforts to defeat your opponents.

One should approach the Treatise from a practical perspective, studying what is in front of us instead of looking for hidden formulas that don't exist. We should first develop and apply what we can understand before trying to delve into the more esoteric aspects of our practices. Unfortunately, as Wang Zongyue said, many would rather seek what they may or may not attain instead of working on what is in front of them. This is the meaning of mistakenly letting go of the near to chase after the far.

As for the statement 捨己從人, letting go of self and flowing with the opponent, there are many levels of interpretations.

People often get confused about the concepts of Adhesion and Yielding, believing that Adhering involves chasing the opponent's hands while Yielding involves moving away from his force. We cannot refer to them as Adhering and Yielding unless they meet Wang Zongyue's definition, which necessitates stagnating the opponent while maintaining Rou, which is to maintaining the unity of Yielding and Adhesion, Yin and Yang.

The second interpretation involves flowing with the opponent and letting his own strength and momentum defeat himself. It is often referred to as 借力打力, borrowing the force to defeat the force. Unless the opponent is completely unskilled, he is not going to willingly commit to issuing force or letting you capitalise on his momentum and weaknesses in his structure. You must therefore deceive him by luring his power out and flowing with him until he defeats himself.

The third interpretation of letting go of yourself and flowing with the opponent is, as taught to me specifically by my teacher, the late grandmaster Wei Shuren in Beijing, about borrowing the opponent's 意氣, his Yi, and his Qi. To help you understand, we will need to approach it from a practical perspective instead of dealing with the more esoteric or spiritual meanings. As Wang Zongyue said, do not let go of the near and chase after the far.

意 Yi

If you cannot understand Yi from a practical perspective, you will never understand the practice of Tai Chi Chuan nor how to borrow Yi Qi. From a martial arts perspective, you can view Yi as mind-intent, thoughts that drive action. For example, if you want to move your hand, no matter how much you think about it, it will never move because that is not Yi. When you are to move your hand, you will first have the intention to do so, and then you will simply move your hands; this is the essence of Yi. When your hand moves without having to think, that is what we call 無意出真意 true-Yi emerging from no-Yi. When you first learn to drive a car, you will need to think about turning, changing gears, how to operate the pedals, and looking at the gauges and reading the road signs. Once you gain experience, all you need is the intention, or Yi, to turning the corner, and your body will perform all the necessary actions to steer the car without effort. Once you are so used to the route, you just need to think of the destination, and you will get there, and that becomes the true-Yi emerging from no-Yi. It is also the 從心所欲, whatever the heart desires, described in (23). These are some examples of different kinds of Yi that you can experience on a daily basis.

氣 **Qi**

The reality of 氣 Qi is a hotly debated subject. Some people hold the belief that Qi is substance, while others dismiss it as mere hot air (pun intended). The concept of Qi is called such because it resembles air—that something is there, but you cannot see it nor feel it unless it is doing something. When we say to infuse the body with Qi or to sink the Qi, it definitely does not mean that you are infusing air or sinking air, although breathing techniques may help you achieve it. In the Wang Zongyue Tai Chi Treatise, he only mentioned Qi once, in sentence (7).

I am not here to argue over the existence or the non-existence of Qi; for all I care, you can call it "X" because names are just labels. One can argue endlessly about the existence or non-existence of Qi, but it remains meaningless until one can practically apply the concepts. Again, don't let go of the near to chase after the far.

From a martial arts perspective, consider Qi as a medium that transmits information and energy from your Yi to both your body and that of your opponent's, causing movements or physiological effects. You can also infuse your weapons and the space around you with Qi. Whether this medium is neural, physical, metaphysical, or a combination of all of them, I have no solid proof, only educated guesses. What matters is not what Qi really is, but rather the application of this concept in martial arts and its role in enhancing human function.

意氣從人借 Borrowing Yi Qi from the Opponent

The practice of Tai Chi is all about 意氣 Yi Qi. There is also a 神 Shen component, and the hierarchy of the Shen Yi Qi command chain is very specific. Since I have extensively discussed this vast subject in my previous publications, I will not delve into it here. I will focus on the aspect of Yi Qi that is relevant to the Treatise.

You should not move your body directly when performing Tai Chi forms, such as the empty-handed or sword forms. Instead, use your Yi to direct your Qi, and your Qi will propel your body or the sword. Some practitioners do the forms by looking at their hands; however, that is not driving the body with Yi Qi; that is just focusing on the hands. Others drive the Qi with the body, but that is incorrect as well, as it should be the Qi driving the body and not the other way around. The purpose of practicing using the Yi Qi to drive the body is to teach the body to obey the Yi Qi and not to move haphazardly on its own. When the entire body moves with Qi, it moves like a wave. It can be subtle like a ripple or powerful like a tsunami.

When you practice the form, you use your own Yi Qi to propel the movement. However, when dealing with an opponent, your mind must be clear, and only your Shen remains. Your techniques are thus driven by the mind-intent of the opponent without interference from your own thoughts and preconceptions. Your body, as you have been teaching it to follow Yi Qi, responds to the opponent's Yi Qi immediately, achieving statement (2) 無過不及，隨曲

就伸, no excess nor deficiencies, comfortably bends and casually extends. Everything must be casual and just right. You are thus achieving 敵未(微)動我先動; before the opponent moves, I move, because you are responding to his mind and not chasing after his actions. Some oral transitions describe it as slight movements, instead of before moving, as the pronunciation for 未 and 微 is very similar; your choice over which one you wish to adopt. In *The Unfettered Mind*, Takuan Soho mentioned "the interval into which not even a hair can be entered," meaning that the responses to the opponent's techniques should be immediate, without a time interval. The only way to respond with such spontaneity and precision is to do it without thoughts. Therefore, by borrowing the opponent's Yi Qi, you are letting go of yourself and flowing with them.

This is the Treatise.